NURTURING LIFE

A First-Time Pregnant Woman's Guide

RUTH PETERS

COPYRIGHT

Copyright © 2023 Ruth Peters

TABLE OF CONTENT

INTRODUCTION

Welcome to the Journey of Motherhood

Congratulations! You stand at the threshold of a remarkable odyssey, a journey unlike any other—a journey of motherhood. Within you, a world unfolds, and with each passing day, you become more intimately connected to the miracle of life. As you embark on this transformative path, know that you are not alone. This guidebook aims to be your faithful companion, your beacon of knowledge and solace, as you navigate the twists and turns of this extraordinary expedition.

Let us depart together, hand in hand, delving into the wondrous mysteries that lie before you. This book seeks to unveil the veils of uncertainty and fill your heart with confidence, as we explore the depths of pregnancy's ebbs and flows. From the subtlest flutter to the resounding drumbeat of your baby's arrival, we shall revel in the symphony of life unfolding within you.

With each page turned, we shall venture into the enigmatic realm of your changing body, where every curve and contour whispers tales of creation. Feel the gentle sway of nature's brush as it paints new hues upon your skin, a canvas of metamorphosis. Together, we shall uncover the secrets of the miraculous vessel that houses this burgeoning life, honoring the profound beauty that resides within your very core.

Our expedition shall continue into the mystical world of your baby's growth, a tapestry woven with the delicate threads of time. From the intricate dance of cells to the awe-inspiring formation of tiny limbs, we shall witness the emergence of a tiny miracle—a life nurtured by your love, and a testament to the wonders of existence itself.

As we traverse the peaks and valleys of this journey, we shall not shy away from the challenges that may arise. Like a ship weathering a tempestuous sea, we shall navigate the turbulence together. Morning sickness, fatigue, and the emotional tempests that sweep through your being—we shall offer counsel and comfort, kindling resilience within your spirit.

The anticipation builds as we approach the shores of labor and delivery—a transformative rite of passage that awaits you. Fear not, for we shall equip you with knowledge, unraveling the mysteries of contractions and stages of labor, empowering you to embrace the raw strength that lies within. Together, we shall prepare a sacred space for your baby's grand entrance, honoring the sacred dance of birth.

This guidebook aims to not only nourish the precious bond between you and your baby but also to nurture your own spirit. We shall encourage the tender petals of self-care to unfurl, reminding you that in the vast tapestry of motherhood, your own well-being is a vital thread. For only when you tend to your own flame can you illuminate the path for your little one.

And as we reach the final pages of this guide, we shall celebrate the splendor of parenthood. We shall revel in the unbreakable ties of family and cherish the memories that etch themselves upon your heart. Our journey may draw to a close, but the echoes of love and wonder shall resound within you, forever etching this chapter into the tapestry of your life.

CHAPTER 1

UNDERSTANDING PREGNANCY STAGES

In the secret embrace of creation, a single spark ignites. As egg and sperm unite, a celestial waltz begins. The stage is set, and the groundwork is laid for the marvelous journey ahead.

A fragile whisper announces the arrival of pregnancy. Deep within, a tiny seed takes root, nestled within the sanctuary of the womb. Like a tender bud, it grows and blossoms, embracing the first stirrings of life. With each passing day, the miracle deepens. Within the sanctuary of your body, a symphony of growth and transformation orchestrates the creation of tiny features and beating heart. Limbs emerge, and the precious form takes shape, bearing the indelible mark of identity.

As the sun climbs higher in the sky, the second trimester dawns, a time of radiant bloom. With the ebbing of morning sickness, energy surges forth. The womb becomes a playground, alive with fluttering movements and joyous kicks. A mother's gentle touch is met with a tender response, forging a connection that transcends words.

As the third trimester commences, anticipation mounts. The crescendo of life resounds within your very being. Your body, a vessel of nurturing, prepares for the grand finale. Braxton Hicks contractions whisper of what lies ahead, reminding you of the strength that resides within.

And then, the long-awaited moment arrives. Like a symphony's climax, the labor of love commences. Contractions ebb and flow, guiding your baby's passage into the world. Time stands still as you harness the depths of your strength, embracing the sacred act of bringing life forth. And in the awe-inspiring crescendo, your little one emerges, bathed in the light of a new beginning.

Within these stages, a woman's body becomes a testament to the incredible power of creation. It is a tapestry woven with love, resilience, and unwavering devotion—a tapestry that binds generations and unfurls the eternal dance of life.

FIRST TRIMESTER OF PREGNANCY

The first trimester of pregnancy, spanning from conception to around week 12, is a remarkable period filled with significant changes and developments for both the baby and the mother. Let's embark on a detailed journey through this transformative phase.

1. The Baby's Development:

   - Week 1-2: Following fertilization, a miraculous fusion of egg and sperm takes place, forming a single-celled entity known as a zygote. The zygote begins its journey down the fallopian tube towards the uterus.

- Week 3-4: Implantation occurs as the zygote attaches itself to the uterine lining. Cells rapidly divide, and the embryo starts to take shape. The primitive structures of the brain, spinal cord, and heart begin to form.

- Week 5-6: The baby's heart starts beating, and blood begins to circulate. Facial features, including eyes, ears, and mouth, start to develop. The neural tube closes, forming the basis for the nervous system.

- Week 7-8: Limb buds emerge, and tiny fingers and toes begin to form. Major organs, such as the liver, kidneys, and lungs, start to develop. The baby's size increases significantly.

- Week 9-10: Facial features become more defined, and the baby starts to exhibit reflex movements. External genitalia also begin to differentiate, although it may not be visible on ultrasound yet.

- Week 11-12: By the end of the first trimester, the baby's vital organs are in place. The baby is about 2.5 to 3 inches long and weighs approximately half an ounce. Facial characteristics continue to develop, and the baby can make subtle movements.

2. Physical Changes in the Mother:

- Hormonal Changes: The mother's body undergoes significant hormonal shifts, particularly an increase in human chorionic gonadotropin (hCG) and progesterone, supporting the pregnancy and preparing the uterus for the baby's growth.

- Morning Sickness: Many women experience nausea, sometimes accompanied by vomiting, commonly known as morning sickness.

This is attributed to hormonal changes and can occur at any time of the day.

   - Breast Changes: Breasts may become tender, swollen, or more sensitive due to increased blood flow and hormonal changes. The areolas may darken, and small bumps called Montgomery's tubercles may appear.

   - Fatigue: The body adapts to pregnancy by increasing blood volume, which can lead to feelings of fatigue and exhaustion. Rest and proper nutrition become crucial during this time.

   - Frequent Urination: As the uterus expands, it puts pressure on the bladder, leading to increased frequency of urination.

   - Emotional Changes: Hormonal fluctuations may contribute to mood swings, ranging from elation to weepiness or irritability. It's important to prioritize self-care and emotional well-being.

3. Medical Care and Support:

   - Prenatal Care: The first trimester is a critical time to seek prenatal care. Regular check-ups, blood tests, and ultrasounds help monitor the baby's development and ensure the mother's well-being.

   - Dietary Considerations: A balanced and nutritious diet, including prenatal vitamins, supports the baby's growth. Certain foods, such as raw or undercooked meats, fish high in mercury, and unpasteurized dairy products, should be avoided.

   - Lifestyle Adjustments: Expectant mothers are often advised to quit smoking, avoid alcohol and recreational drugs, and limit caffeine intake to ensure a healthy environment for the baby.

- Emotional Support: Pregnancy can bring a range of emotions. Seeking support from loved ones, joining prenatal classes, or connecting with support groups can provide reassurance and valuable guidance

The first trimester is a time of awe-inspiring beginnings, where the foundation for your baby's growth is laid. It's a period of immense change and adaptation for the mother. By embracing proper care, nurturing oneself, and relishing the wonders of this transformative phase, both mother and baby set forth on a remarkable journey of love and discovery.

SECOND TRIMESTER OF PREGNANCY

The second trimester of pregnancy, spanning from weeks 13 to 28, is often referred to as the "honeymoon phase" of pregnancy. During this time, both the baby and the mother undergo remarkable developments and experiences. Let's delve into the details of this extraordinary period.

1. Baby's Development:

   - Week 13-16: Your baby experiences rapid growth. Facial features become more refined, and tiny fingerprints start forming. The baby's bones continue to develop, and the gender may be detectable through ultrasound.

   - Week 17-20: Your baby's movements become more noticeable, and you may start feeling gentle flutters known as "quickening." Fine hair, called lanugo, covers the baby's body to regulate body temperature. The baby's skin thickens and becomes less translucent.

- Week 21-24: Eyebrows and eyelashes appear, and the baby's senses continue to develop. The lungs undergo essential maturation, preparing for breathing outside the womb. The baby's kicks and movements become stronger.

- Week 25-28: The baby's brain experiences rapid growth, and the neural connections strengthen. Eyes open and close, and the baby may respond to external sounds and light. Fat stores begin to accumulate, providing insulation and energy for the baby's growth.

2. Physical Changes in the Mother:

- Growing Belly: As the baby grows, your belly expands noticeably. You may start to show a prominent baby bump, bringing excitement and a visible reminder of the miracle within.

- Increased Energy: Many women experience a surge of energy during the second trimester, as morning sickness subsides and the body adjusts to pregnancy.

- Relief from Discomforts: Common discomforts such as nausea, breast tenderness, and frequent urination often diminish or disappear during this phase. However, new challenges may arise, such as backaches and round ligament pain due to the expanding uterus.

- Skin Changes: Some women develop a pregnancy "glow," with improved skin tone and texture. However, hormonal changes can also cause skin pigmentation changes, including darkened patches or a linea nigra (a dark vertical line on the abdomen).

- Weight Gain: A steady and healthy weight gain becomes more apparent during the second trimester. It is essential to follow your healthcare provider's guidance to ensure optimal well-being for both you and your baby.

3. Milestones and Exciting Moments:

- Feeling Baby's Movements: As your baby grows stronger, you will experience more pronounced movements. These gentle flutters or kicks are a beautiful connection between you and your baby.

- Gender Reveal: If you choose, the second trimester is a time when the baby's gender may be determined through an ultrasound. It can be an exciting moment to share with loved ones.

- Bonding with Baby: As your baby's senses develop, talking, singing, and gentle touch can create a deep bond between you and your little one. They can recognize familiar voices and respond to external stimuli.

4. Preparation and Care:

- Prenatal Check-ups: Regular prenatal appointments continue during the second trimester. These visits monitor your health and ensure the baby's growth and development are on track.

- Prenatal Tests: Your healthcare provider may recommend specific tests, such as a mid-pregnancy ultrasound (anatomy scan) to assess the baby's growth and detect any potential issues.

- Exercise and Nutrition: Staying active with exercises approved by your healthcare provider promotes overall well-being. A balanced diet rich in nutrients is crucial for your baby's development.

- Childbirth Education: The second trimester is an ideal time to consider childbirth education classes, where you can learn about labor, delivery, and coping

Techniques.

- Emotional Wellness: Taking care of your emotional well-being is essential. Communicate with your support system, express any concerns, and seek professional help if needed.

The second trimester is a period of blossoming, where the awe-inspiring presence of your growing baby becomes more tangible. Cherish the precious moments, prioritize self-care, and savor this phase as you journey towards the final trimester, awaiting the joyous arrival of your little one.

THIRD TRIMESTER OF PREGNANCY

The third trimester of pregnancy, which spans from week 29 until the birth of your baby, is a time of anticipation and preparation for the final stretch of your pregnancy journey. Let's explore the significant aspects and experiences of this transformative period.

1. Baby's Development:

- Week 29-32: Your baby's growth continues, and they start to fill out and gain weight. Organs mature further, and the bones harden. The baby's brain continues to develop rapidly.

- Week 33-36: Your baby's movements may feel more limited as they occupy a larger space within the womb. They settle into a head-down position, preparing for birth. The baby's immune system strengthens, acquiring antibodies from you.

- Week 37-40+: At full term, your baby is ready for birth. They continue to gain weight, adding more fat layers for insulation and nourishment after birth. Their organs are fully developed, and they are prepared for life outside the womb.

2. Physical Changes in the Mother:

- Growing Belly: Your belly expands even further, and you may feel the weight and size of your baby more prominently. It can affect your posture and balance.

- Braxton Hicks Contractions: You may experience Braxton Hicks contractions, which are practice contractions that help prepare the uterus for labor. They are usually irregular and not as intense as true labor contractions.

- Increased Discomfort: As your baby grows and puts pressure on your organs, you may experience increased discomfort, such as heartburn, shortness of breath, backaches, and swollen feet and ankles.

- Frequent Urination: The pressure on your bladder intensifies, leading to more frequent trips to the bathroom.

- Fatigue: The physical demands of carrying a growing baby can cause fatigue, making it important to prioritize rest and sleep.

3. Nesting and Preparations:

- Baby's Nursery: The third trimester is a time to set up your baby's nursery, creating a cozy and safe space for their arrival. Decorating, organizing baby essentials, and washing baby clothes can be exciting tasks.

- Birth Plan: Discuss and finalize your birth plan with your healthcare provider. This plan outlines your preferences for labor, pain management, and other aspects of childbirth.

- Packing Hospital Bag: Prepare a bag with essentials for your hospital stay, including clothes for you and the baby, toiletries, and necessary documents.

- Infant CPR and Newborn Care Classes: Consider attending classes that cover topics like infant CPR and newborn care. They can provide valuable knowledge and boost your confidence as you prepare to care for your baby.

4. Emotional Rollercoaster:

- Mixed Emotions: The anticipation of meeting your baby may be accompanied by a mix of excitement, joy, anxiety, and even a touch of nervousness. It's normal to experience a range of emotions during this time.

- Bonding with Baby: As you near the end of your pregnancy, continue to bond with your baby through talking, singing, and gentle touch. Respond to their movements and establish a connection that will deepen after birth.

- Support System: Lean on your support system for emotional support and practical assistance. Share your feelings, concerns, and joys with loved ones, friends, or support groups.

5. Final Check-ups and Preparations:

- Prenatal Visits: Your healthcare provider will schedule regular prenatal check-ups to monitor your health and the baby's well-being. These visits may become more frequent as you approach your due date.

- Baby Position and Labor Preparation: Your healthcare provider will monitor your baby's position and assess their readiness for birth. They may discuss the signs of labor and offer guidance on what to expect.

- Birth Classes: Consider attending childbirth education classes to learn about the stages of labor, pain management options, breathing techniques, and partner support during delivery.

The third trimester marks the final stage of your pregnancy, bringing you closer to the momentous arrival of your baby. Embrace the physical changes, prepare your mind and surroundings, and cherish this unique time as you eagerly await the joyous birth of your little one.

PRENATAL CARE AND CHECKUPS

In the sacred dance of pregnancy, prenatal care emerges as a harmonious symphony, weaving together the intricate threads of nurturing and safeguarding both mother and baby. Each note, a tender touchpoint, guides expectant mothers through a transformative journey of care and support. Let us explore the essence of prenatal care in a unique and enchanting style.

As the dawn of pregnancy breaks, the journey of prenatal care commences. A melody of anticipation fills the air, leading expectant mothers to their first prenatal checkup. Here, amidst the gentle hum of medical instruments and the soothing lullaby of a healthcare provider's voice, a profound connection forms. They weave a tapestry of trust, as stories are shared, and concerns are gently embraced.

In the subsequent movements of prenatal care, a rhythmic cadence emerges. Like the ebb and flow of a serene river, expectant mothers find solace in regular checkups, each visit an opportunity to listen to the life within. With each passing appointment, the melodic harmony of the baby's heartbeat resonates, a reassuring affirmation of their well-being.

Prenatal care unfolds as a pas de deux between the expectant mother and her healthcare provider. Together, they navigate the intricacies of growth. With gentle hands, measurements are taken, mapping the baby's progress and ensuring a symmetrical dance of development. The mother's expanding belly becomes a canvas, where the artistry of life is painted with love and meticulous attention.

In the embrace of prenatal care, knowledge blossoms like delicate petals. Education becomes a lyrical melody, guiding expectant mothers through the intricacies of pregnancy. The healthcare provider's voice, like a soothing lullaby, shares wisdom about nutrition, exercise, and self-care. Together, they explore the nuances of labor and birth, empowering the mother to embark upon this transformative journey with confidence.

The rhythm of prenatal care reverberates beyond the confines of the clinic walls. It becomes a harmonious ensemble, comprising not only the expectant mother and her healthcare provider but also the chorus of loved ones and support systems. Partners, family, and friends join the symphony, attending appointments, lending listening ears, and embracing the expectant mother's journey. Their presence adds depth and resonance, fortifying the melody of care.

As the final movements of pregnancy draw near, the crescendo of prenatal care swells. In these moments, expectant mothers find solace in the meticulous monitoring, ensuring a smooth transition into the grand finale of birth. The healthcare provider's gentle guidance and unwavering support create a safe haven where the expectant mother can surrender to the rhythm of labor, knowing she is enveloped in a web of care and expertise.

Within the tapestry of prenatal care, expectant mothers discover not only medical guidance but also a sanctuary of compassion and connection. It is a journey of nurturing, where the expectant mother and her healthcare provider engage in a graceful duet, orchestrating the harmonious symphony of pregnancy. In this unique style, the magic of prenatal care unfolds, weaving the intricate threads of love and support, resonating with the tender beauty of new life.

NURTURING EMOTIONAL WELL BEING

In the enchanting realm of pregnancy, the nurturing of emotional well-being blooms as a delicate blossom, requiring tender care and attention. Within the transformative journey of creating life, expectant mothers are encouraged to embark on an inner voyage, embracing the depths of their emotions with compassion and love.

As the seeds of life take root, a symphony of emotions begins to play. The expectant mother finds herself immersed in a myriad of feelings, from joy and excitement to moments of vulnerability and uncertainty. Amidst the whirlwind of pregnancy, cultivating inner stillness becomes an oasis for the expectant mother's emotional well-being. Like a calm lake reflecting the moon's gentle glow, moments of solitude and self-reflection offer respite from the external noise. Through mindfulness practices, meditation, or simply connecting with nature, the expectant mother finds solace in the serenity of her own being.

Just as a delicate flower requires nourishment and care, the expectant mother must tend to her emotional landscape. This may involve setting boundaries, seeking support from loved ones, or engaging in activities that bring joy and fulfillment. By recognizing and embracing her emotional needs, the expectant mother creates a sanctuary of self-compassion.

Like vibrant hues on a painter's canvas, expressive arts and therapeutic practices offer a unique avenue for emotional expression and exploration. Through creative outlets such as journaling, painting, dance, or music, the expectant mother taps into her inner reservoir of emotions, giving voice to the depths of her being. These artistic journeys become a cathartic release, fostering emotional well-being and self-discovery. In moments when the emotional landscape feels overwhelming, seeking professional support becomes an empowering choice.

Just as a garden flourishes with attentive nurturing, the expectant mother tends to her own well-being with love and kindness. This may involve nourishing the body with wholesome foods, engaging in gentle exercise, prioritizing restful sleep, and indulging in activities that replenish the spirit.

Within the realm of pregnancy, nurturing emotional well-being becomes an essential art form, intertwining with the creation of life itself. By embracing the symphony of emotions, cultivating inner stillness, honoring emotional needs, fostering connection, exploring expressive arts, seeking support, and prioritizing self-care, the expectant mother embraces the transformative power of emotional well-being. May this unique and heartfelt guide serve as a gentle companion on this remarkable journey, illuminating the path towards emotional nourishment and serenity.

CHAPTER 2

CHANGES IN YOUR BODY

During the mesmerizing voyage of pregnancy, a woman's body undergoes a miraculous transformation, like a sculptor's masterpiece evolving with each passing day. From the gentle swell of the belly to the nurturing embrace of maternal curves, these physical changes weave a tapestry of life. Let us embark on a journey through the enchanting realm of physical transformations during pregnancy, painted with vivid brushstrokes of description.

The Blossoming Bump

As the seed of life takes root, a subtle transformation begins. The abdomen, once flat and taut, becomes a sacred canvas where the miracle of creation unfolds. With each passing week, the gentle swell of the belly becomes more pronounced, cradling the growing life within like a protective cocoon. It is a breathtaking sight, a testament to the profound beauty of motherhood.

The Curves of Creation

The breasts, once soft and supple, swell with nourishing milk, embracing their maternal purpose. The hips widen, creating a generous space for the growing life within. These curves become a celebration of femininity and strength, a testament to the body's magnificent ability to nurture new life.

A Symphony of Sensations

As pregnancy progresses, a symphony of sensations accompanies the physical changes. The expectant mother may feel the flutter of tiny kicks, like delicate butterfly wings caressing her womb. She may experience the stretching of ligaments, reminding her of the miraculous expansion taking place within. Each sensation, from gentle movements to subtle aches, becomes a reminder of the life blossoming within her.

The Radiance of Glow

Pregnancy unveils a radiant glow that emanates from within. Like a soft halo of light, it envelops the expectant mother, enhancing her natural beauty. The skin becomes more luminous, imbued with a subtle blush. A sparkle dances in her eyes, reflecting the awe and anticipation of the life she carries. This radiant glow becomes a testament to the joy and vitality that accompanies the journey of motherhood.

The Symphony of Breathing

As the baby grows, the expectant mother's body adapts to accommodate the expanding life within. The lungs, like gentle bellows, work in harmony with the body, ensuring a steady flow of oxygen to both mother and baby. The rhythm of breath becomes a constant companion, a reminder of the extraordinary connection between the two intertwined souls.

The Dance of Balance

In the delicate dance of pregnancy, the body adjusts to maintain balance and harmony. The center of gravity shifts, encouraging the expectant mother to move with grace and intention. As her body nurtures new life, she discovers newfound strength and agility, adapting to the changes with resilience and grace. The dance of balance becomes a testament to the body's remarkable ability to adjust and support the growing life within.

The physical transformations of pregnancy are a testament to the awe-inspiring miracle of creation. From the blossoming bump to the curves of creation, each change is a testament to the body's remarkable ability to nurture and sustain life. May this vivid exploration of physical transformations during pregnancy serve as a celebration of the extraordinary beauty that accompanies this transformative Journey.

COMMON DISCOMFORTS AND HOW TO MANAGE THEM

Pregnancy is a beautiful journey, but it can also bring about certain discomforts. Here are some common discomforts during pregnancy and tips on managing them:

1. Nausea and Morning Sickness:

   - Eat small, frequent meals throughout the day to avoid an empty stomach.

   - Avoid spicy, greasy, and fatty foods that may trigger nausea.

   - Ginger, lemon, or peppermint can help alleviate nausea.

   - Stay hydrated by drinking plenty of fluids.

2. Fatigue and Low Energy:

   - Prioritize rest and sleep. Take short naps during the day if needed.

   - Maintain a balanced diet and include foods rich in iron and folate.

   - Engage in gentle exercises like walking or prenatal yoga to boost energy levels.

3. Backache and Body Pains:

   - Practice good posture while sitting and standing.

   - Wear comfortable, supportive shoes.

   - Use pillows for added support while sleeping.

   - Apply a warm compress or take a warm bath to ease muscle tension.

   - Consider prenatal massages or chiropractic care (after consulting your healthcare provider).

4. Frequent Urination:

   - Avoid drinking excessive fluids before bedtime.

   - Empty your bladder completely when urinating.

   - Wear loose and comfortable clothing that doesn't put pressure on your bladder.

5. Heartburn and Indigestion:

   - Eat small, frequent meals instead of large ones.

   - Avoid spicy, greasy, and acidic foods.

   - Sit upright while eating and for a while after meals.

   - Consider raising the head of your bed to prevent nighttime heartburn.

6. Swollen Feet and Ankles:

   - Elevate your legs whenever possible.

   - Avoid standing or sitting for long periods.

   - Wear comfortable, supportive shoes.

   - Regularly perform gentle foot exercises and ankle rotations.

7. Constipation:

- Eat a high-fiber diet with plenty of fruits, vegetables, and whole grains.

   - Drink ample water and fluids.

   - Engage in regular physical activity, such as walking.

   - Talk to your healthcare provider before taking any over-the-counter laxatives.

8. Varicose Veins and Leg Cramps:

   - Avoid standing or sitting for long periods.

   - Elevate your legs when resting.

   - Wear compression stockings to support blood circulation.

   - Stretch your legs and calf muscles before bedtime.

   - Increase your potassium intake with foods like bananas and spinach.

Remember, every pregnancy is unique, and it's essential to consult with your healthcare provider about any discomforts you experience. They can provide personalized advice and recommendations based on your specific needs. Enjoy this special time and take care of yourself.

CHAPTER 3

NAVIGATING PREGNANCY CHALLENGES

HORMONAL CHANGES AND MOOD SWINGS

Pregnancy involves a significant increase in hormone production, which can lead to various physical and emotional changes. Hormonal fluctuations during pregnancy can have an impact on your mood, causing mood swings. Understanding these changes can help you cope better. Here's what you need to know:

During pregnancy, your body experiences increased levels of hormones such as estrogen and progesterone. These hormones play crucial roles in supporting the growth and development of the baby. However, they can also influence your emotional state.

Mood swings are common during pregnancy and are often attributed to hormonal changes. You may find yourself feeling elated and joyful one moment, then suddenly becoming tearful or irritable the next. These mood swings can be unpredictable and may vary in intensity.

Hormonal changes alone may not be solely responsible for mood swings. Factors such as fatigue, stress, physical discomfort, changes in body image, and anticipation of motherhood can also contribute to emotional ups and downs.

While it's normal to experience mood swings during pregnancy, there are ways to manage and alleviate them:

- Practice self-care: Prioritize activities that help you relax and unwind, such as taking a warm bath, engaging in gentle exercise, or practicing mindfulness or meditation.

- Seek support: Talk openly with your partner, family, or friends about your feelings. Sharing your emotions and concerns can provide comfort and understanding.

- Stay connected: Join prenatal support groups or online communities where you can connect with other expectant mothers who may be going through similar experiences.

- Get enough rest: Fatigue can exacerbate mood swings, so ensure you're getting adequate sleep and rest throughout the day.

- Maintain a healthy lifestyle: Eating a well-balanced diet, staying hydrated, and engaging in regular physical activity can positively influence your mood.

- Communicate with your healthcare provider: If you're experiencing severe mood swings or emotional difficulties that interfere with your daily life, don't hesitate to reach out to your healthcare provider. They can offer guidance and support.

Remember, mood swings during pregnancy are normal and typically subside after childbirth. However, if you're concerned about your emotional well-being or notice persistent feelings of sadness or anxiety, it's important to seek professional help.

DEALING WITH COMMON PREGNANCY COMPLICATIONS

Here's some information about common complications in pregnancy, along with tips on how to avoid them and manage them if they arise:

1. Gestational Diabetes:

Gestational diabetes is a type of diabetes that develops during pregnancy. It is characterized by high blood sugar levels that occur for the first time during pregnancy and typically resolves after childbirth.

During pregnancy, the body naturally becomes more resistant to insulin, a hormone that helps regulate blood sugar levels. In some cases, the pancreas may not be able to produce enough insulin to overcome this resistance, leading to elevated blood sugar levels and the development of gestational diabetes.

Gestational diabetes can pose risks to both the mother and the baby if not properly managed. It increases the chances of certain complications during pregnancy and delivery, such as high blood pressure, preeclampsia, and the need for cesarean section. Additionally, the baby may be at a higher risk of excessive birth weight, low blood sugar levels after birth, and an increased likelihood of developing type 2 diabetes later in life.

To manage gestational diabetes, a healthcare provider typically recommends the following:

1. Blood sugar monitoring: Regularly checking blood sugar levels throughout the day using a glucose meter.

2. Healthy eating: Following a well-balanced meal plan that includes a variety of foods, with a focus on complex carbohydrates, lean proteins, and healthy fats. Monitoring portion sizes and spreading meals and snacks throughout the day are also important.

3. Regular physical activity: Engaging in moderate-intensity exercise as advised by a healthcare provider, such as walking or swimming, to help lower blood sugar levels and improve insulin sensitivity.

4. Medication, if needed: In some cases, insulin injections or oral medications may be prescribed to help manage blood sugar levels.

It's important to note that gestational diabetes can usually be managed effectively with proper medical care, diet, and exercise. With appropriate management, most women with gestational diabetes give birth to healthy babies. After delivery, blood sugar levels usually return to normal, but women who have had gestational diabetes have a higher risk of developing type 2 diabetes later in life, so ongoing monitoring of blood sugar levels is important.

2. Preterm Labor:

Preterm labor refers to the onset of regular contractions and cervical changes that occur before the 37th week of pregnancy. It is important to be aware of the signs and symptoms of preterm labor so that you can take appropriate action. Here's what you need to know:

1. Signs and Symptoms:

   - Contractions: Regular contractions that occur every 10 minutes or more frequently.

   - Pelvic pressure: A feeling of increased pressure or heaviness in the pelvis.

   - Low backache: Persistent or intermittent pain or discomfort in the lower back.

   - Abdominal cramping: Cramps similar to menstrual cramps, with or without diarrhea.

   - Vaginal discharge: An increase in vaginal discharge or a change in its consistency.

   - Fluid leakage: Fluid leaking from the vagina, which may indicate ruptured membranes (water breaking).

2. Risk Factors:

   While preterm labor can happen to any pregnant woman, certain factors may increase the risk:

   - Previous preterm birth.

   - Multiple pregnancies (twins, triplets, etc.).

- Certain uterine or cervical abnormalities.

- Infections during pregnancy.

- Smoking, substance abuse, or high levels of stress.

- Short time period between pregnancies.

- Chronic conditions like high blood pressure or diabetes.

3. When to Seek Medical Help:

If you experience any signs or symptoms of preterm labor, it's important to contact your healthcare provider immediately. They can assess your condition and provide guidance. It's better to be safe and seek medical attention promptly, as early intervention can significantly improve outcomes.

4. Managing Preterm Labor:

If you are diagnosed with preterm labor, your healthcare provider may recommend various interventions, depending on the specific situation. These may include:

- Medications: Your provider may prescribe medications, such as corticosteroids, to help mature the baby's lungs and reduce the risk of complications.

- Bed rest: In some cases, modified bed rest or restricted activity may be advised to decrease stress on the uterus.

- Monitoring: Your healthcare provider will closely monitor your condition, including fetal well-being and contractions, through regular check-ups and tests.

- Hospitalization: Severe cases of preterm labor may require hospitalization for closer monitoring and specialized care.

5. Prevention:

While it's not always possible to prevent preterm labor, there are steps you can take to reduce the risk:

- Attend prenatal check-ups regularly.

- Avoid smoking, substance abuse, and excessive alcohol consumption.

- Eat a healthy, balanced diet and stay adequately hydrated.

- Manage chronic conditions and infections appropriately.

- Minimize stress and seek support when needed.

Remember, every pregnancy is unique, and the management of preterm labor will depend on individual circumstances. It's important to maintain open communication with your healthcare provider, follow their advice, and report any concerns promptly.

3. High blood pressure and Pre-eclampsia

High blood pressure, also known as hypertension, is a condition characterized by elevated blood pressure levels. When high blood pressure develops during pregnancy, it is referred to as gestational hypertension. However, if it is accompanied by organ damage and other complications, it may be diagnosed as pre-eclampsia.

1. Gestational Hypertension:

Gestational hypertension is high blood pressure that develops after the 20th week of pregnancy. It typically resolves after childbirth. It is important to monitor and manage gestational hypertension to avoid complications.

2. Pre-eclampsia:

Pre-eclampsia is a condition characterized by high blood pressure and signs of damage to organs such as the liver and kidneys. It usually develops after the 20th week of pregnancy and can affect both the mother and the baby. If left untreated, pre-eclampsia can lead to serious complications.

Signs and Symptoms of Pre-eclampsia:

It's important to be aware of the signs and symptoms of pre-eclampsia, which can include:

- High blood pressure (140/90 mmHg or higher)

- Severe headaches

- Vision changes, such as blurred vision or seeing spots

- Abdominal pain, especially in the upper right side

- Swelling, particularly in the hands, face, or legs

- Sudden weight gain (more than 2 pounds per week)

Managing High Blood Pressure and Pre-eclampsia:

If you develop high blood pressure or pre-eclampsia during pregnancy, your healthcare provider will closely monitor your condition and may recommend the following:

1. Regular Prenatal Check-ups:

   Attend all scheduled prenatal appointments to monitor your blood pressure, urine protein levels, and overall health.

2. Medications:

   In some cases, medication may be prescribed to help lower blood pressure and manage pre-eclampsia. Your healthcare provider will determine the most appropriate medication for you and closely monitor its effects.

3. Lifestyle Modifications:

   Follow your healthcare provider's recommendations regarding diet, exercise, and weight management. Reduce sodium intake, increase water consumption, and eat a balanced diet with plenty of fruits, vegetables, and whole grains.

4. Rest and Relaxation:

   Get plenty of rest and avoid excessive physical exertion. Take breaks throughout the day and prioritize self-care.

5. Monitoring Fetal Well-being:

Regular monitoring of the baby's growth, movements, and heart rate will be conducted to ensure their well-being. This may involve ultrasounds, non-stress tests, or other specialized tests.

6. Delivery:

Depending on the severity of pre-eclampsia and the gestational age of the baby, early delivery may be necessary to prevent complications. Your healthcare provider will determine the optimal timing and mode of delivery.

If you experience any signs or symptoms of pre-eclampsia or have concerns about your blood pressure, it is important to contact your healthcare provider immediately. They will be able to assess your condition, provide appropriate management, and ensure the best possible outcome for you and your baby.

6. Anemia

Anemia is a condition characterized by a decrease in the number of red blood cells or a decrease in the amount of hemoglobin in the blood. During pregnancy, anemia is relatively common and can occur due to various factors. It is important to understand anemia in pregnancy and how to manage it effectively. Here's what you need to know:

1. Causes of Anemia in Pregnancy:

Anemia in pregnancy can be caused by:

- Increased blood volume: The volume of blood in your body increases during pregnancy, which can dilute the concentration of red blood cells.

- Iron deficiency: Iron is essential for the production of red blood cells. Inadequate iron intake or poor absorption can lead to iron-deficiency anemia.

- Folate deficiency: Folate (also known as folic acid) is crucial for red blood cell production. Inadequate folate intake can contribute to anemia.

- Vitamin B12 deficiency: Vitamin B12 is necessary for the production of healthy red blood cells. Deficiency can lead to anemia.

2. Symptoms of Anemia:

Anemia during pregnancy may present with the following symptoms:

- Fatigue and weakness

- Pale skin and nails

- Shortness of breath

- Rapid or irregular heartbeat

- Dizziness or lightheadedness

- Difficulty concentrating

3. Diagnosis:

Anemia is diagnosed through a blood test that measures hemoglobin levels. Your healthcare provider may also assess other parameters related to red blood cells and iron stores.

4. Prevention and Management:

To prevent and manage anemia during pregnancy, consider the following strategies:

- Iron-rich diet: Consume foods rich in iron such as lean meats, poultry, fish, legumes, dark green leafy vegetables, and fortified grains.

- Iron supplementation: Your healthcare provider may prescribe iron supplements if your iron levels are low or if you are at risk of developing anemia.

- Folate and vitamin B12 intake: Ensure an adequate intake of foods containing folate and vitamin B12, such as leafy greens, citrus fruits, fortified cereals, and dairy products.

- Prenatal vitamins: Take prenatal vitamins as prescribed by your healthcare provider, as they typically contain iron, folate, and other essential nutrients.

- Iron absorption enhancers: Consume iron-rich foods with vitamin C-rich foods (e.g., citrus fruits) to enhance iron absorption.

- Avoid iron inhibitors: Avoid consuming tea, coffee, and calcium-rich foods within one to two hours of consuming iron-rich foods, as they can hinder iron absorption.

- Follow healthcare provider's advice: Attend regular prenatal check-ups and follow your healthcare provider's recommendations for managing anemia.

5. Monitoring:

Your healthcare provider will monitor your hemoglobin levels throughout pregnancy to ensure they are within a healthy range. Follow-up blood tests may be conducted to assess the effectiveness of any interventions or treatments.

If you suspect you may have anemia or have any concerns about your symptoms, it's important to consult with your healthcare provider for proper diagnosis and guidance. They can provide personalized advice based on your individual circumstances.

Remember, maintaining adequate nutrition, especially iron, folate, and vitamin B12, is crucial during pregnancy to prevent and manage anemia. With appropriate management, most cases of anemia during pregnancy can be effectively addressed.

DANGER SIGNS IN PREGNANCY

During pregnancy, it is important to be aware of certain danger signs that may indicate potential complications. Recognizing these signs and seeking prompt medical attention is crucial for ensuring the well-being of both the expectant mother and the baby. In this discussion, we will explore some common danger signs in pregnancy that warrant immediate medical attention.

1. Vaginal Bleeding: Any amount of vaginal bleeding during pregnancy should be taken seriously and reported to a healthcare provider. It may indicate conditions such as placental abruption, miscarriage, or preterm labor.

2. Severe or Persistent Abdominal Pain: Intense or persistent abdominal pain that is unrelated to normal pregnancy discomforts should be evaluated by a healthcare professional. It may indicate conditions like ectopic pregnancy, appendicitis, or preeclampsia.

3. Severe Headaches: Severe or persistent headaches accompanied by visual disturbances, dizziness, or high blood pressure can be signs of preeclampsia or other underlying issues. Immediate medical attention is necessary.

4. Sudden or Excessive Swelling: While mild swelling is common in pregnancy, sudden or excessive swelling of the hands, face, or legs can be indicative of preeclampsia or other conditions. It should be evaluated by a healthcare provider.

5. Reduced Fetal Movement: If the baby's movements significantly decrease or cease altogether, it is important to seek medical attention immediately. Reduced fetal movement may indicate fetal distress or other complications.

6. Signs of Preterm Labor: Any signs of preterm labor, such as regular contractions before 37 weeks, lower back pain, pelvic pressure, or a change in vaginal discharge, should be addressed promptly to prevent premature birth.

7. Leakage of Fluid: If there is a sudden gush or a continuous trickle of fluid from the vagina, it may indicate the rupture of membranes. This could lead to infection or premature labor, requiring immediate medical assessment.

8. Severe Nausea and Vomiting: While nausea and vomiting are common in pregnancy, severe and persistent symptoms could be signs of conditions like hyperemesis gravidarum, which require medical attention to prevent dehydration and complications.

9. High Fever: A persistent high fever during pregnancy may be a sign of infection, which can be harmful to both the mother and the baby. Medical evaluation is essential to identify and treat the underlying cause.

10.   Signs of Deep Vein Thrombosis (DVT): Symptoms such as swelling, pain, warmth, or redness in the legs can be indicative of DVT, a blood clot in the deep veins. DVT during pregnancy requires immediate medical attention to prevent potentially life-threatening complications.

It is important for expectant mothers to familiarize themselves with these danger signs and to promptly report any concerns to their healthcare provider. Regular prenatal care and open communication with medical professionals are vital for early detection, diagnosis, and appropriate management of any potential complications. Remember, it is always better to seek medical advice and have peace of mind rather than ignoring a potential danger sign.

The management of danger signs in pregnancy depends on the specific complication or condition being experienced. However, in general, it is crucial to take the following steps when encountering any danger sign during pregnancy:

1. Contact Your Healthcare Provider: If you experience any of the identified danger signs, reach out to your healthcare provider immediately. Describe your symptoms or concerns in detail and follow their instructions for further evaluation and management.

2. Follow Medical Advice: Once you have communicated with your healthcare provider, carefully follow their guidance. They may recommend coming in for an examination, advising specific tests or diagnostic procedures to determine the cause of the symptoms.

3. Seek Emergency Care if Necessary: In some cases, danger signs may indicate a more urgent situation. If you are experiencing severe symptoms such as heavy bleeding, intense pain, difficulty breathing, or loss of consciousness, it is important to seek emergency medical care without delay. Call emergency services or go to the nearest emergency room.

4. Adhere to Treatment Plans: Depending on the diagnosis, your healthcare provider will create an individualized treatment plan. It may include medications, lifestyle modifications, bed rest, dietary changes, or other interventions. It is essential to adhere to the prescribed treatment plan to manage the condition effectively.

5. Attend Regular Follow-ups: Regular prenatal care appointments are crucial throughout pregnancy, especially if you have experienced any danger signs. These appointments allow your healthcare provider to monitor your condition, assess the well-being of you and your baby, and make any necessary adjustments to your care plan.

6. Seek Emotional Support: Experiencing danger signs in pregnancy can be stressful and emotionally challenging. It is important to seek emotional support from your partner, loved ones, or healthcare professionals. They can provide reassurance, understanding, and guidance to help you navigate any concerns or anxieties.

Remember, every pregnancy is unique, and the management of danger signs will vary based on individual circumstances. Trust in the expertise of your healthcare provider and communicate openly with them about your symptoms and concerns. Prompt action and early intervention can often lead to better outcomes for both you and your baby.

CHAPTER 4

COMMON PREGNANCY CONCERN

DIET IN PREGNANCY

A healthy and balanced diet during pregnancy is essential for the growth and development of both you and your baby. It's important to consume a variety of nutritious foods to meet the increased nutritional needs during this time. Here are some key points to consider:

1. Macronutrients:

  - Carbohydrates: Choose whole grains, fruits, vegetables, and legumes to provide energy, fiber, and essential nutrients.

  - Proteins: Include lean meats, poultry, fish, eggs, dairy products, legumes, and plant-based protein sources like tofu and quinoa to support tissue growth and repair.

  - Healthy fats: Opt for sources like avocados, nuts, seeds, and olive oil, which provide essential fatty acids and fat-soluble vitamins.

2. Micronutrients:

- Folate: Consume foods rich in folate, such as leafy greens, citrus fruits, fortified cereals, and legumes, to help prevent birth defects.

   - Iron: Include iron-rich foods like lean meats, poultry, fish, fortified cereals, spinach, and dried fruits to support red blood cell production.

   - Calcium: Ensure sufficient intake of dairy products, fortified plant-based milk alternatives, leafy greens, and calcium-fortified foods for strong bones and teeth.

   - Vitamin D: Get exposure to sunlight and consume vitamin D-rich foods like fatty fish, fortified dairy products, and egg yolks to support calcium absorption.

   - Omega-3 fatty acids: Include sources like fatty fish (e.g., salmon, sardines), walnuts, chia seeds, and flaxseeds for brain and eye development.

3. Hydration:

   Drink plenty of fluids, especially water, throughout the day to support healthy digestion, circulation, and hydration.

4. Food Safety:

   - Avoid raw or undercooked meats, seafood, and eggs to reduce the risk of foodborne illnesses.

   - Minimize consumption of high-mercury fish (e.g., shark, swordfish, king mackerel) and limit caffeine intake.

- Wash fruits and vegetables thoroughly, and practice good hygiene in food preparation to prevent contamination.

5. Small, Frequent Meals:

Instead of large meals, aim for smaller, more frequent meals and snacks to manage digestion, reduce heartburn, and stabilize blood sugar levels.

6. Healthy Snacking:

Choose nutritious snacks such as fruits, vegetables with hummus or yogurt dip, nuts, seeds, whole-grain crackers, or homemade smoothies.

7. Prenatal Supplements:

Take a prenatal vitamin and mineral supplement as recommended by your healthcare provider to ensure adequate intake of essential nutrients.

8. Individual Needs and Restrictions:

Consider any specific dietary requirements or restrictions you may have and consult with your healthcare provider or a registered dietitian for personalized guidance.

Maintaining a healthy diet during pregnancy is not about eating for two, but rather about making nutrient-dense choices to support your own health and the growth and development of your baby. Focus on quality over quantity and listen to your body's hunger and fullness cues.

USE OF DRUGS

When it comes to the use of drugs during pregnancy, it's crucial to approach the topic with caution and prioritize the safety of both the mother and the developing baby. Here's some important information to consider:

1. Medications and Substances:

   - Prescription Medications: Inform your healthcare provider about any prescription medications you are taking. They can assess the risks and benefits and determine if any adjustments or alternative options are necessary.

   - Over-the-Counter Medications: Some over-the-counter medications may be safe to use during pregnancy, but it's essential to consult with your healthcare provider or pharmacist before taking them, as not all are suitable for pregnant women.

   - Herbal Remedies and Supplements: Certain herbal remedies and dietary supplements may not be safe during pregnancy. Always consult with your healthcare provider before using any herbal or dietary supplements.

- Illicit Drugs and Recreational Substances: Illicit drugs and recreational substances should be strictly avoided during pregnancy, as they can pose significant risks to both the mother and the baby.

2. Risks and Benefits:

Each medication or substance carries its own risks and benefits. Your healthcare provider will consider factors such as the specific drug, dosage, duration of use, and the stage of pregnancy to assess potential risks to the developing baby. They will weigh these risks against the potential benefits of using the medication to make an informed decision.

3. Communication with Healthcare Provider:

Open and honest communication with your healthcare provider is essential. Inform them about any medications, substances, or supplements you are taking or considering taking, even if they are not prescription medications. This includes disclosing any history of substance abuse or addiction.

4. Teratogenicity:

Some medications are known to be teratogenic, meaning they can cause birth defects or developmental abnormalities. It's important to discuss the potential risks with your healthcare provider and explore alternative treatment options when available.

5. Pregnancy Category System:

Medications are often classified into pregnancy categories to provide guidance on their use during pregnancy:

- Category A: Considered safe for use during pregnancy based on studies.

- Category B: Generally considered safe, but more research may be needed.

- Category C: Use with caution, as potential risks are uncertain.

- Category D: Potential risks are known, but in certain situations, the benefits may outweigh the risks.

- Category X: Contraindicated during pregnancy due to significant risks.

6. Proper Use of Medications:

If medications are prescribed during pregnancy, follow your healthcare provider's instructions carefully. Take the prescribed dosage and duration as advised. Do not modify or discontinue any medication without consulting your healthcare provider first.

SEX DURING PREGNANCY

Sexual activity and intimacy can be a normal and healthy part of many pregnancies. However, it's important to consider a few factors and take certain precautions. Here are some key points to keep in mind:

1. Communication with Your Partner:

   Open and honest communication with your partner is crucial. Discuss your feelings, concerns, and any discomfort you may experience. This will help both of you understand each other's needs and make adjustments if necessary.

2. Physical Changes and Comfort:

   As your pregnancy progresses, you may experience physical changes that can affect your comfort during sexual activity. These changes may include breast tenderness, fatigue, increased vaginal discharge, and changes in libido. Listen to your body and communicate your comfort levels with your partner.

3. Positions:

   Experiment with different positions to find what works best for you and your partner. You may find that certain positions alleviate discomfort or provide more comfort and support during intercourse. Consider positions that allow you to control the depth and pace of penetration.

4. Pelvic Floor Exercises:

   Engaging in pelvic floor exercises, such as Kegel exercises, can help strengthen the muscles that support the pelvic organs. This may enhance sexual satisfaction and help with postpartum recovery.

5. Safety Precautions:

While sex is generally safe during a healthy pregnancy, there are a few situations when you should exercise caution:

- If you have a history of preterm labor or other complications, consult your healthcare provider for guidance.

- Avoid sexual activity if you have a ruptured amniotic sac (water breaking), vaginal bleeding, or if your healthcare provider has advised against it.

- Use protection (e.g., condoms) to reduce the risk of sexually transmitted infections (STIs) if there is a potential exposure.

6. Emotional Well-being:

Pregnancy can bring about a range of emotions, including changes in body image and heightened anxiety. Emotional intimacy and connecting with your partner outside of sexual activity are just as important as physical intimacy. Communicate your feelings, offer support, and prioritize emotional connection.

7. Consult with Your Healthcare Provider:

If you have any concerns or specific medical conditions, it's advisable to consult with your healthcare provider. They can provide personalized guidance based on your individual circumstances.

ACTIVITY AND EXERCISE

Staying active and engaging in regular exercise during pregnancy is generally beneficial for both you and your baby. However, it's important to approach exercise with caution and make adjustments based on your individual circumstances. Here are some key points to consider:

1. Consult with Your Healthcare Provider:

Before starting or continuing an exercise routine, consult with your healthcare provider. They can assess your overall health and provide personalized guidance based on your medical history, current pregnancy, and any specific considerations.

2. Benefits of Exercise during Pregnancy:

Regular exercise during pregnancy can offer numerous benefits, such as:

- Increased stamina and strength for labor and delivery.

- Improved mood and reduced risk of prenatal depression.

- Enhanced circulation and reduced risk of varicose veins.

- Better weight management and improved body image.

- Reduced pregnancy discomforts like back pain and constipation.

- Improved sleep quality.

3. Suitable Activities:

Choose low-impact exercises that are gentle on your joints and accommodate your growing belly. Suitable activities may include:

- Walking: A simple and accessible exercise that can be done throughout pregnancy.

- Swimming: Provides buoyancy and supports your weight, relieving pressure on joints.

- Prenatal yoga or Pilates: Focuses on flexibility, strength, and relaxation.

- Prenatal aerobics or dance classes: Specifically designed for pregnant women.

- Stationary cycling: Provides a low-impact cardiovascular workout.

4. Exercise Guidelines:

Keep the following guidelines in mind when exercising during pregnancy:

- Warm-up: Start each session with a gentle warm-up to prepare your body for exercise.

- Stay hydrated: Drink plenty of water before, during, and after exercise to prevent dehydration.

- Wear comfortable clothing: Choose loose-fitting, breathable attire and supportive shoes.

- Listen to your body: Pay attention to any discomfort, dizziness, or shortness of breath. Modify or stop exercising if needed.

- Pelvic floor exercises: Include pelvic floor exercises, such as Kegels, to strengthen the pelvic muscles.

- Avoid lying flat on your back: After the first trimester, avoid exercises that involve lying flat on your back for extended periods, as it may restrict blood flow to the uterus.

5. Exercise Precautions:

While exercise is generally safe during pregnancy, take precautions to ensure your safety:

- Avoid high-impact activities or contact sports that may carry a risk of injury or falls.

- Modify exercises as your pregnancy progresses to accommodate your changing body.

- If you have any medical conditions or complications, follow your healthcare provider's advice regarding exercise limitations.

6. Postpartum Exercise:

After delivery, gradually resume exercise based on your healthcare provider's guidance. Allow your body time to heal before engaging in more intense activities.

Every pregnancy is unique, and it's important to listen to your body and make adjustments as needed. If you experience any pain, excessive fatigue, vaginal bleeding, or have concerns, contact your healthcare provider for guidance.

BABY SHOPPING

Baby shopping for a pregnant woman can be an exciting and joyful experience as she prepares for the arrival of her baby. Here are some considerations and tips for baby shopping

1. Create a checklist: Start by making a checklist of essential items that the baby will need. This can include clothing, bedding, feeding supplies, diapers, and other necessary items. It will help you stay organized and ensure that you don't forget anything important.

2. Maternity clothing: As your body undergoes changes during pregnancy, comfortable and well-fitting clothing becomes essential. Look for maternity clothes that are designed to accommodate a growing belly and provide comfort. This includes maternity jeans, tops, dresses, bras, and underwear.

3. Baby essentials: Purchase essential items like a crib, mattress, changing table, and dresser. Ensure that these items meet safety standards and are durable. Consider the space available in the nursery and choose furniture accordingly.

4. Clothing and accessories: Buy a range of clothing for the baby, including onesies, sleepers, socks, hats, and mittens. Opt for soft, breathable fabrics that are gentle on the baby's skin. It's also a good idea to have a few outfits in different sizes since babies grow quickly.

5. Feeding supplies: If the you plan to breastfeed, consider purchasing nursing bras, breast pads, and a breast pump. If you intend to bottle-feed, buy bottles, nipples, bottle sterilizers, and formula. Nursing pillows can also be helpful for comfortable feeding sessions.

6. Diapering essentials: Stock up on diapers, wipes, diaper rash creams, and diaper bags. It's a good idea to have diapers in different sizes to accommodate the baby's growth. Consider buying a changing pad or a changing table to make diaper changing more convenient.

7. Baby care and hygiene: Purchase baby bath products, including gentle soap, shampoo, lotion, and washcloths. Invest in a baby bathtub or a bath seat for safe and comfortable bathing experiences.

8. Maternity and nursing essentials: Consider your needs as well. Maternity pillows, supportive bras, comfortable sleepwear, and nursing pads can enhance your comfort during pregnancy and breastfeeding.

9. Safety and health items: Buy baby-proofing supplies such as outlet covers, cabinet locks, baby gates, and corner protectors to ensure a safe environment for the baby. Additionally, a thermometer, nasal aspirator, and a basic first aid kit can come in handy for addressing the baby's health needs.

10. Baby registry: Consider setting up a baby registry to share with family and friends. This allows them to contribute to the items you need and reduces the chances of receiving duplicate gifts.

CHAPTER 5

PREPARING FOR LABOR AND DELIVERY

CREATING A BIRTH PLAN

Creating a birth plan can help you communicate your preferences and expectations for your birthing experience to your healthcare provider and support team. Here's a step-by-step guide on how to create a birth plan:

1. Gather Information:

Educate yourself about the different options and procedures available during labor and delivery. Attend childbirth education classes, read reputable books or articles, and have discussions with your healthcare provider. Understanding your choices will help you make informed decisions.

2. Choose Your Birth Setting:

Decide where you want to give birth. Options include a hospital, birthing center, or home birth. Consider the level of medical intervention available, your comfort level, and any specific preferences you may have.

3. Determine Your Support Team:

Decide who you want to have by your side during labor and delivery. This may include your partner, a family member, or a doula. Discuss their roles and responsibilities in supporting your birth preferences.

4. Outline Your Preferences:

Write down your preferences for various aspects of labor and delivery. Some common considerations include:

- Labor environment: Specify your preferences for lighting, music, privacy, and any comfort measures you would like to have, such as a birthing ball or a tub for water immersion.

- Pain management: Outline your preferred pain management techniques, whether you prefer natural coping techniques, pharmacological pain relief options, or a combination.

- Labor positions: Mention any specific labor positions you prefer, such as walking, squatting, or using a birthing chair.

- Monitoring and interventions: State your preferences regarding fetal monitoring, episiotomy, induction, or assisted delivery methods such as forceps or vacuum extraction.

- Delivery preferences: Specify whether you want to have an active role in pushing, the use of a mirror to view the birth, or if you would like to have immediate skin-to-skin contact with your baby.

- Cesarean birth: If you have any preferences or concerns regarding a cesarean birth, outline them in your birth plan.

- Postpartum preferences: Include preferences for breastfeeding, newborn procedures, and whether you would like to have your baby in the room with you at all times.

5. Discuss with Your Healthcare Provider:

Share your birth plan with your healthcare provider during prenatal visits. Review it together, discuss any medical considerations, and ensure that your preferences align with the available options and any specific circumstances.

6. Communicate with Your Support Team:

Share your birth plan with your partner, family members, and doula, if applicable. Make sure they understand your preferences and can advocate for you during labor and delivery.

7. Be Flexible:

Keep in mind that birth plans can serve as a guide, but it's important to remain flexible. Labor and delivery can be unpredictable, and circumstances may require adjustments to the plan to prioritize the safety and well-being of you and your baby.

8. Review and Revise:

Regularly review and revise your birth plan as needed. As your pregnancy progresses, your preferences or medical circumstances may change. Update your birth plan accordingly and communicate any updates with your healthcare provider and support team.

A birth plan is a tool to express your preferences, but it's important to maintain open communication with your healthcare provider and remain flexible during the birthing process. Their expertise and guidance will ensure the best possible outcomes for you and your baby.

Here are some common birth plan options that you can consider including in your birth plan:

1. Labor Environment:

   - Lighting preferences: Specify whether you prefer dimmed lights or natural lighting.

   - Music or sound preferences: State whether you would like to have your own music playlist or other sounds playing during labor.

   - Privacy preferences: Indicate your desire for privacy during labor and whether you want limited staff presence.

2. Pain Management:

- Natural coping techniques: Mention your preferences for using breathing exercises, relaxation techniques, movement, massage, or hydrotherapy for pain relief.

- Pharmacological pain relief: Outline your preferences for specific pain relief options, such as nitrous oxide, IV medications, epidural anesthesia, or a combined spinal-epidural.

3. Labor Positions:

- Specify your preferred labor positions, such as walking, squatting, using a birthing ball, or utilizing a birthing chair.

- Mention any positions you would like to avoid or have reservations about.

4. Fetal Monitoring and Interventions:

- Fetal monitoring preferences: Specify your preferences for intermittent or continuous fetal monitoring during labor.

- Episiotomy: State your preference regarding episiotomy (surgical incision to enlarge the vaginal opening) and whether you prefer it to be avoided unless medically necessary.

- Induction and augmentation: If you have preferences regarding labor induction or augmentation (stimulation of contractions), include them in your birth plan.

5. Delivery Preferences:

- Pushing preferences: Mention your desire to actively participate in pushing or to follow your body's cues.

- Mirror use: Indicate whether you would like to have a mirror available to view the birth.

- Immediate skin-to-skin contact: State if you want to have immediate skin-to-skin contact with your baby after delivery.

6. Cesarean Birth Preferences:

- Specify your preferences for cesarean birth if it becomes necessary, such as a gentle cesarean approach, delayed cord clamping, or having a support person present in the operating room.

- Skin-to-skin contact: Mention your preference for having skin-to-skin contact with your baby in the operating room or recovery area.

7. Postpartum Preferences:

- Breastfeeding: Indicate your desire to breastfeed and whether you would like assistance with initiating breastfeeding soon after delivery.

- Newborn procedures: Specify your preferences regarding newborn procedures like eye ointment, Vitamin K injection, or cord blood banking.

- Rooming-in: State whether you want your baby to stay with you in the room at all times or if you prefer nursery care at specific times.

These options may vary depending on the birthing facility, healthcare provider, and any specific medical circumstances. It's important to discuss these preferences with your healthcare provider and understand what is feasible and safe for you and your baby.

Customize your birth plan based on your personal preferences and values, while keeping in mind that flexibility may be necessary depending on the course of your labor and any unexpected circumstances that may arise.

BIRTH SETTING OPTIONS

Here are the common birth setting options to consider when planning for your childbirth:

1. Hospital Birth:

   - Hospital births are the most common birth setting and offer access to medical interventions, technology, and a team of healthcare professionals.

   - Hospitals provide specialized care for high-risk pregnancies or medical complications that may require immediate medical attention during labor and delivery.

   - In hospitals, you have access to pain management options, such as epidurals and other pharmacological pain relief methods.

   - Hospitals typically have operating rooms available for emergency cesarean births if needed.

- Some hospitals offer options for natural birthing environments within the hospital setting, such as birthing suites or rooms with amenities like birthing tubs, low lighting, and comfortable furnishings.

2. Birthing Center:

   - Birthing centers are designed to provide a more homelike and low-intervention setting for childbirth.

   - They offer a comfortable and less clinical environment compared to hospitals.

   - Birthing centers are typically staffed by midwives or nurse-midwives who focus on supporting natural childbirth and promoting a personalized experience.

   - They often provide options for water births, natural pain management techniques, and minimal medical interventions.

   - Birthing centers may have partnerships with nearby hospitals in case of emergencies or the need for a transfer during labor.

3. Home Birth:

   - Home births involve giving birth in the comfort of your own home, supported by a qualified midwife or certified professional.

   - Home births are generally recommended for low-risk pregnancies and women who desire a natural and intimate birthing experience.

   - With home births, you have the freedom to create a personalized environment and have more control over the entire birthing process.

- Midwives attending home births are trained to handle emergency situations and carry necessary equipment and medications.

- It's important to have a thorough discussion with your healthcare provider and midwife to ensure that you are a suitable candidate for a home birth and to establish a plan for transfer to a hospital if needed.

When choosing a birth setting, it's essential to consider your individual preferences, medical history, and any potential risk factors. Discuss your options with your healthcare provider and consider factors such as access to emergency medical care, availability of pain management options, and your comfort level with medical interventions.

Take note, the safety and well-being of you and your baby should be the primary consideration when deciding on a birth setting. Make an informed decision based on your unique circumstances and desires, and ensure you have a skilled and qualified healthcare provider or midwife to support you throughout the birthing process.

THE HOSPITAL DELIVERY BAG

Preparing a hospital delivery bag is an essential task for a pregnant woman as you approache your due date. Here are some tips on how to prepare a hospital delivery bag:

1. Start early: Begin preparing your hospital delivery bag a few weeks before your due date to ensure you have everything ready in case of an early arrival.

2. Essentials for labor and delivery:

- Identification and hospital paperwork: Bring your identification, health insurance information, and any necessary hospital registration or admission forms.

- Birth plan: If you have a birth plan, include a copy in your bag to share with your healthcare providers.

- Comfortable clothing: Pack loose and comfortable clothes for labor and recovery. This can include a loose-fitting nightgown or a nursing gown, a robe, slippers, and comfortable underwear. Don't forget to pack nursing bras if you plan to breastfeed.

- Toiletries: Include items like a toothbrush, toothpaste, shampoo, conditioner, body wash, and a hairbrush. Lip balm and lotion can also be helpful for dry skin.

- Snacks and drinks: Pack some light and energy-boosting snacks like granola bars, nuts, and dried fruits. Also, consider bringing your own water bottle or preferred beverages.

- Entertainment: Labor can be a lengthy process, so consider bringing items to keep you occupied, such as books, magazines, a tablet, or music playlists.

3. Postpartum essentials:

- Comfortable clothing: Pack loose, comfortable clothes for the postpartum period, such as maternity leggings, loose tops, and comfortable underwear. Don't forget to pack maternity pads or disposable adult diapers for post-birth bleeding.

- Nursing supplies: If you plan to breastfeed, include nursing pads, nipple cream, and a breastfeeding pillow.

- Toiletries: Include your regular toiletries like a toothbrush, toothpaste, shampoo, conditioner, body wash, and a hairbrush.

- Going-home outfit: Choose a comfortable and loose outfit to wear when you leave the hospital. Make sure it accommodates any postpartum belly size.

4. Other essentials:

- Baby clothes and essentials: Pack a few outfits for the baby, including onesies, sleepers, socks, and a hat. Additionally, bring receiving blankets, diapers, wipes, and a baby blanket.

- Car seat: Make sure the car seat is properly installed in your vehicle. You'll need it to safely transport your baby home from the hospital.

- Electronics and chargers: Don't forget to pack your phone, camera, or any other electronic devices you may want to capture special moments. Bring chargers for these devices as well.

5. Miscellaneous items:

- Important documents: Carry important documents like your ID, health insurance information, and your partner's contact information.

- Cash and change: Keep some cash and change on hand for parking fees or vending machines.

- Contact list: Have a list of important phone numbers, including your healthcare provider and emergency contacts.

It will be important to check with your healthcare provider or the hospital for any specific items they recommend or provide. Keep the bag easily accessible, and communicate with your partner or support person about where it is stored. Packing your hospital delivery bag in advance can help reduce stress and ensure you have everything you need for a smooth and comfortable stay at the hospital during labor and recovery.

SIGNS OF LABOR TO LOOK OUT FOR

As a pregnant woman, it is essential to be aware of the signs of labor to recognize when your body is preparing for childbirth. Here are some common signs of labor to look out for:

1. Regular and increasing contractions: Contractions are the tightening and relaxing of the uterine muscles. True labor contractions become more regular, intense, and closer together over time. They typically last for around 30 to 70 seconds and occur at intervals that gradually shorten. Unlike Braxton Hicks contractions

(which are usually irregular and less intense), true labor contractions continue regardless of your activity level or changes in position.

2. Bloody show: A few days or hours before labor, you might notice a small amount of blood-tinged mucus called the "bloody show." This is the result of the cervix thinning and dilating in preparation for labor.

3. Rupture of membranes (water breaking): The amniotic sac surrounding the baby can rupture, leading to a gush or a slow trickle of fluid from the vagina. This is commonly referred to as the "water breaking." If your water breaks, it's important to contact your healthcare provider to inform them, even if you're not experiencing contractions yet.

4. Backache and pelvic pressure: As labor approaches, you may experience increased backache and intense pressure in the pelvic area. This can be a result of the baby's head engaging in the pelvis, getting ready for birth.

5. Cervical changes: Your healthcare provider can perform cervical checks to assess changes in the cervix. As labor nears, the cervix will start to efface (thin out) and dilate (open up). However, it's important to note that cervical changes can happen gradually and may not always be an accurate predictor of when labor will begin.

6. Increased vaginal discharge: As labor approaches, you may notice an increase in vaginal discharge. It can be thicker and pinkish or brownish in color.

7. Nesting instinct and burst of energy: Some women experience a burst of energy and a strong nesting instinct shortly before going into labor. This may manifest as an intense desire to clean, organize, or prepare for the baby's arrival.

It's important to note that not all signs of labor occur in the same order or with the same intensity for every woman. Some signs may be more subtle or may not occur until labor is well underway. If you experience any signs or have concerns about labor, it's essential to contact your healthcare provider to discuss your symptoms and receive appropriate guidance.

Remember, each pregnancy is unique, and the signs of labor can vary. Staying informed, attending prenatal appointments, and maintaining open communication with your healthcare provider will help you navigate the labor process with confidence.

When labor begins, it's important to keep certain dos and don'ts in mind to ensure a safe and comfortable experience. Here are some guidelines to consider:

Dos:

1. Do stay calm and relaxed: Labor can be an intense and challenging experience, but maintaining a calm and relaxed mindset can help manage pain and facilitate the progress of labor. Practice deep breathing, visualization, and other relaxation techniques learned during childbirth education classes.

2. Do time your contractions: Monitor the duration, frequency, and intensity of your contractions. Time the length of each contraction and the time between contractions. This information can help you determine when to reach out to your healthcare provider and when it's time to go to the hospital or birthing center.

3. Do communicate with your healthcare provider: Keep in touch with your healthcare provider throughout the process. Inform them about the onset of labor, the progression of contractions, and any changes in your water breaking or other significant symptoms.

4. Do change positions: Experiment with different positions to find the most comfortable one during labor. Walking, rocking on a birthing ball, leaning forward on a bed or chair, or kneeling on all fours can help ease discomfort and facilitate labor progress.

5. Do stay hydrated: Sip on water, clear fluids, or isotonic drinks to stay hydrated during labor. It's important to maintain your energy levels and prevent dehydration.

6. Do utilize pain management techniques: Depending on your birth plan and preferences, consider utilizing pain management techniques such as breathing exercises, massage, relaxation techniques, water therapy (if available), or other methods recommended by your healthcare provider.

7. Do listen to your body: Pay attention to your body's cues and follow your instincts. Trust your body's ability to birth and communicate your needs to your healthcare provider and birth support team.

Don'ts:

1. Don't panic: Remember that labor is a natural process, and panicking can increase stress levels and hinder progress. Stay focused, breathe deeply, and trust in your body's ability to give birth.

2. Don't delay contacting your healthcare provider: If you notice any concerning symptoms or your healthcare provider has advised you to contact them under specific circumstances, don't hesitate to reach out. They are there to guide and support you throughout the labor process.

3. Don't engage in strenuous activities: As labor progresses, avoid engaging in strenuous physical activities that could exhaust you or potentially compromise your safety or the baby's well-being.

4. Don't eat heavy meals: During active labor, it's generally advised to stick to light snacks and clear fluids rather than consuming heavy meals. This helps prevent discomfort and potential complications if a medical intervention becomes necessary.

5. Don't forget to pack and bring essentials: Ensure you have your hospital delivery bag prepared in advance and bring it with you when heading to the hospital or birthing center. This includes essential items for both you and your baby, as well as important documents and contact information.

6. Don't hesitate to ask for support: Surround yourself with a supportive birth team, which can include your partner, family members, a doula, or healthcare professionals. Don't hesitate to ask for support, whether it's physical, emotional, or informational.

Know this, every labor experience is unique, and it's important to follow the guidance of your healthcare provider and the specific protocols and practices of your chosen birthing facility. Trust in yourself and your support system, and embrace the journey of bringing your baby into the world.

STAGES OF LABOR

Understanding the stages of labor is crucial for expectant mothers and their partners as they prepare for the childbirth journey. Labor is a complex process that occurs in distinct stages, each serving a specific purpose in bringing the baby into the world. In this discussion, we will explore the three stages of labor in detail, including the signs, duration, and key events that occur during each stage.

Stage 1: Early Labor

Early labor, also known as the latent phase, marks the beginning of the labor process. This stage is characterized by mild and irregular contractions, which gradually increase in frequency, duration, and intensity. Here's a breakdown of the different phases within Stage 1:

1. Early Phase: During this phase, the cervix begins to efface (thin out) and dilate (open). Contractions may be irregular, lasting around 30-60 seconds and occurring every 5-20 minutes. The expectant mother may experience backache, mild discomfort, and a bloody show, which is the release of a small amount of mucus and blood from the cervix.

2. Active Phase: As labor progresses, contractions become more frequent, longer, and stronger. The cervix continues to dilate, reaching around 6 centimeters or more. Contractions typically occur every 3-5 minutes and last for 45-60 seconds. The expectant mother may feel increased pressure in the pelvic area, and discomfort intensifies.

3. Transition Phase: This is the final phase of Stage 1 and often the most intense. Contractions become extremely strong, lasting around 60-90 seconds and occurring every 2-3 minutes. The cervix fully dilates to 10 centimeters. The expectant mother may experience a sense of urgency, restlessness, nausea, and an increased desire to push.

Stage 2: Active Labor and Delivery

Stage 2 marks the onset of active labor and the actual delivery of the baby. During this stage, the cervix is fully dilated, and the expectant mother begins to push with each contraction. Key events in Stage 2 include:

1. Pushing Phase: The expectant mother actively participates by pushing with each contraction to help move the baby through the birth canal. The contractions may become less frequent but more intense. The healthcare provider guides and supports the mother during this phase, assisting with perineal support and providing guidance on effective pushing techniques.

2. Birth of the Baby: With each push, the baby's head gradually emerges, followed by the rest of the body. The healthcare provider may suction the baby's mouth and nose to clear any fluids and ensure proper breathing. Once the baby is born, the umbilical cord is clamped and cut, and the newborn is placed on the mother's chest for skin-to-skin contact.

Stage 3: Delivery of the Placenta

After the baby is born, there is a final stage known as the delivery of the placenta. This stage is relatively short and involves the detachment and expulsion of the placenta from the uterus. Here's an overview of what occurs:

1. Placental Separation: Following the birth of the baby, contractions continue, aiding in the separation of the placenta from the uterine wall. The healthcare provider monitors the mother for any signs of excessive bleeding or complications.

2. Expulsion of the Placenta: Once the placenta has detached, the healthcare provider guides the mother to push gently to deliver the placenta. This typically occurs within 5-30 minutes after the birth of the baby. The healthcare provider ensures that the entire placenta and membranes are intact to minimize the risk of infection.

Understanding the stages of labor empowers expectant mothers and their partners to prepare for the journey ahead.

It is important to note that labor experiences can vary, and each stage may progress at a different pace for different individuals. Remaining flexible, staying informed, and having a supportive healthcare team can help navigate the stages of labor with confidence and positivity.

PAIN MANAGEMENT OPTION

Here's some information to help educate you about pain management options during labor:

1. Natural Coping Techniques:

Many women choose to use natural coping techniques to manage pain during labor. These techniques include:

- Breathing exercises: Focus on slow, deep breathing to help you relax and manage pain.

- Relaxation techniques: Practice techniques like guided imagery, visualization, or progressive muscle relaxation to promote a sense of calm.

- Movement and positions: Changing positions, walking, rocking, or using a birthing ball can help relieve discomfort and encourage progress in labor.

- Massage and counter-pressure: Gentle massage or applying pressure to specific areas can provide relief and reduce tension.

- Warm water therapy: Immersing yourself in a warm bath or using a birthing pool can help relax your muscles and ease pain.

2. Support from a Birth Partner or Doula:

Having a trusted birth partner or a doula by your side can provide emotional support and offer comfort measures during labor. They can assist with relaxation techniques, massage, and help advocate for your needs.

3. Pharmacological Pain Relief:

There are various pharmacological pain relief options available during labor. It's essential to discuss these options with your healthcare provider in advance to understand their benefits, risks, and potential side effects. Some common pharmacological pain relief options include:

- Nitrous oxide: Also known as "laughing gas," it can be self-administered during contractions to provide temporary pain relief.

- Intravenous (IV) medication: Medications, such as opioids or analgesics, can be administered through an IV to help manage pain. These may cause drowsiness and can affect the baby's alertness after birth.

- Epidural anesthesia: A regional anesthesia technique that involves placing a catheter in the lower back to administer pain relief medication continuously. It provides pain relief while allowing you to remain awake and actively participate in labor. An epidural may slightly increase the duration of labor and may require additional interventions, such as continuous monitoring of the baby's heart rate.

- Combined spinal-epidural: This technique combines the immediate pain relief of a spinal block with the continuous pain relief of an epidural.

4. Knowledge and Birth Preparation:

Attend childbirth education classes or workshops to learn about labor, pain management techniques, and the available options. Understanding the process of labor and being well-informed about your choices can help you feel more empowered and confident during the birthing experience.

5. Individualized Plan:

Every woman's experience and pain tolerance are unique. Discuss your preferences and pain management options with your healthcare provider well in advance of your due date. They can help create an individualized birth plan that takes into account your specific needs, medical history, and any potential contraindications.

Remember, the goal of pain management during labor is to help you cope with the discomfort and create a positive birthing experience. It's important to remain flexible and open to adjusting your pain management plan as labor progresses.

CONCLUSION

In the closing chords of this wondrous journey, we arrive at the conclusion of our exploration into the realm of pregnancy. Throughout these pages, we have embarked on a unique and heartfelt voyage, weaving together knowledge, insights, and a touch of magic to guide first-time pregnant women on their path towards motherhood.

In the tapestry of pregnancy, we have celebrated the stages of growth, marveling at the miraculous transformations occurring within both mother and baby. From the tender beginnings of the first trimester to the blossoming beauty of the second, and the eagerly awaited arrival of the third, we have witnessed the incredible journey of life unfolding.

We have delved into the realms of physical and emotional well-being, embracing the body's changes, nurturing the spirit, and fostering a deep connection between mother and child. From understanding the importance of prenatal care and emotional well-being to exploring comfort measures and managing common discomforts, we have strived to provide guidance, support, and encouragement every step of the way.

Through the chapters on pain management, creating a birth plan, and addressing potential complications, we have empowered expectant mothers to make informed decisions, advocate for their desires, and approach their birth experience with confidence and grace. We have shed light on the importance of collaboration with healthcare providers, the power of support systems, and the art of flexibility in navigating the unpredictable nature of childbirth.

In the realm of self-care and nurturing, we have offered a tapestry of practices and rituals that honor the beauty and sacredness of this transformative time. From cultivating mindfulness and creating nurturing spaces to embracing self-care rituals and nourishing the body, we have encouraged expectant mothers to prioritize their well-being, fostering a foundation of love and resilience.

As we reach the final brushstrokes of this guidebook, let us remember that every pregnancy journey is as unique as the individual traversing it. The wisdom shared within these pages is a gentle compass, guiding and illuminating the path ahead. However, it is the expectant mothers themselves who will infuse their own experiences, dreams, and desires, bringing their own vibrant colors and melodies to the symphony of pregnancy.

May this guidebook be a cherished companion, offering solace, inspiration, and guidance as expectant mothers embrace the sacred journey of bringing new life into the world. May it serve as a reminder of their strength, resilience, and the immense love that flows through every fiber of their being. And may the bonds nurtured during this transformative time continue to blossom and flourish, creating a tapestry of love and connection that weaves through generations to come.

With open hearts and boundless joy, we bid farewell to this exploration, knowing that the journey of motherhood has only just begun. May it be filled with blessings, growth, and an abundance of love as you embark on this remarkable adventure.